The Doorway to Optimal Health and Well Being

Frank J. Door, D.C.

Disclaimer

The information in this book is intended for educational and informational use only and should not be construed as medical advice. The reader should consult with their physician before attempting any activity or making any lifestyle changes discussed in this book. Although every attempt is made to ensure the accuracy of the information presented, the author and publisher are not liable for any illness or injury that may result from attempting any activities or lifestyle changes presented in this book.

ISB 10: 1983941549
ISBN 13: 978-1983941542

Dedication

To everyone who wants good health...naturally.

The Doorway
to Optimal Health
and Well Being

Frank J. Door, D.C.

Introduction

I was raised in a very unconventional family. I was born while my father was attending Palmer Chiropractic College in Davenport Iowa and I received my first adjustment at the tender age of three days old by B.J. Palmer (who you will read about later). My father was the second chiropractor in Puyallup and my mother owned the very first health food store. When one of my family became ill, it was chiropractic adjustments and vitamins as the treatment, while everyone else was going to the medical doctor and getting a vaccination, a flu shot or a prescription for medication. Quite the abnormal family when it came to the treatment of disease and illness.

These days everyone is looking for a quick fix, a super pill, a great new medicine or a cure all drug for any condition that ails you. That is a nice dream, but today's new super drug is tomorrow's latest lawsuit. Remember, every medication that has ever been recalled by the FDA was once deemed safe by the same FDA committee. Think about that the next time you take a prescription drug or an over-the-counter medication. Every day you can pick up a magazine or read on the internet about a new superior drug with a laundry list of side effects. A three page ad in a magazine has two pages of warnings about the terrible side effects; headaches, vomiting, diarrhea, strokes and possible death to name a few. Why would anyone even think about taking these drugs?

Today, people are more receptive to "alternative care" such as chiropractic, vitamins and natural foods, pure bottled water, massage, acupuncture, and more. People are more pro-active in taking care of themselves and asking many more questions. People are tired of the same old message; "here's a prescription for the latest anti-biotic or pain reliever or muscle relaxers or..." They know that message doesn't work anymore. People are tired of pills, potions and lotions with deadly side effects. They want something more. Something natural without harmful side effects. Something that will help their condition and help prevent it from coming back and keep them healthy. They want Chiropractic!

It all starts with The Big Idea.

Table of Contents

Chapter 1

The Big Idea

A slip on the snowy sidewalk is a small thing. It happens to millions.

A fall from a ladder in the summer is a small thing. It also happens to millions.

The slip or fall produces a subluxation. The subluxation is a small thing.

The subluxation produces pressure on a nerve. That pressure is a small thing.

That decreased flowing produces a diseased body and brain. That is a big thing to that man.

Multiply that sick man by a thousand, and you control the physical and mental welfare of a city.

Multiply that man by one hundred thirty million, and you forecast and can prophesy the physical and mental status of a nation.

Now comes a man. And one man is a small thing.

This man gives an adjustment. The adjustment is a small thing.

The adjustment replaces the subluxation. That is a small thing.

The adjusted subluxation releases pressure upon nerves. That is a small thing.

The released pressure restores health to a man. This is a big thing to that man.

Multiply that well man by a thousand, and you step up the physical and mental welfare of a city.

Multiply that well man by a million, and you increase the efficiency of a state.

Multiply that well man by a hundred thirty million, and you have produced a healthy, wealthy, and better race for posterity.

So, the adjustment of the subluxation to release pressure upon nerves, to restore mental impulse flow, to restore health, is big enough to rebuild the thoughts and actions of the world.

The idea that knows the cause, that can correct the cause of disease, is one of the biggest ideas known. Without it, nations fall; with it, nations rise.

This idea is the biggest I know of.

B.J. Palmer, 1944

Chapter 2

The Good Doctor Door

My neck and back were aching,
I could not bend to the floor,

A good friend quickly sent me,
To a chiropractor whose name is Door!

I worried so about going,
I knew he would break me in two,

But the aches and pains were hurting,
So what else could I do?

He snapped and cracked and twisted,
Though I hasten to explain,

In spite of the snapping and cracking,
I didn't feel any pain!

So if you've really got problems,
And you don't want them anymore,

Why don't you get up the courage,
And go see the good Doctor Door!

Chapter 3

The Four BIG Questions

Almost every new patient that comes into a chiropractic office has the same four major questions on their minds:

What is wrong with me?

The simplest, non-medical explanation I can give you is that you have a subluxation (which is a bone out of place in your neck or back), pinching and stretching a nerve, causing pain symptoms, which results in an unhealthy painful condition. No amount of pills, potions or lotions will correct this problem. They may cover up your problems, and you may think it is better, but it is not.

Therefore, in order for you to be healthy and pain-free, the subluxation must be corrected to be in place with no pressure on your nerves.

So, when a friend or family member asks you what is wrong with you, all you have to do is tell them: "I have a bone out of place, pinching a nerve, causing my health problems."

Can you help me?

If your health problem is a result of a bone out of place, pinching a nerve, and causing painful symptoms, then yes, I can help you. Gently returning your spinal bones to their normal position so that you can regain your health is my job.

If your health problem is caused by something other than "a bone out of place" (arthritic bone spurs, bulging discs, etc.) then I will refer you for further examination with another specialist. This may included your primary care physician, massage therapists, nutritionists, physical therapists, neurologists or even surgeons. We will do whatever it takes to help you achieve your health care goals.

How long will it take to get well?

How long it takes depends upon how severe your health problem is, and ho long you have had your symptoms. I offer two treatment options at my office, and you can choose the one that is best for your.

The first treatment option is to "patch" your health problem. The goal of this treatment plan is to just get you out of pain as quickly as possible. It is similar to putting a band-aid on your health problem. This program usually takes several office visits over a two week period.

The second treatment option is to "fix" your health problem (or get it to as near normal as possible). This treatment option offers longer lasting results, and it normally takes several more office visits over a 2-3 month period. At the end of this time period you will be re-evaluated and you may be

done, almost done, or ready for periodic
maintenance care.

How much will it cost?

If you are using your health insurance or
Medicare, you are responsible for any amounts not
paid by your insurance company (deductibles and
co-payments). I am under contract with many
insurance companies to accept their payment as
"payment in full" after your yearly deductible is
met. Your insurance company may be one of these,
and you will not be billed for any unpaid amounts.

If you are injured at work, your employer's
Worker's Compensation insurance policy covers
you 100%. If you are injured in an automobile
accident, the Personal Injury Protection (PIP)
portion of your automobile policy usually pays
100%.

Chapter 4

Questions and Answers

What is Chiropractic?

Chiropractic is the largest non-medical and drug-less form of health care in the world today. Chiropractic is a branch of the healing arts which is based upon the understanding that good health depends on a normally functioning nervous system. It is very important to understand that chiropractic is not a treatment for diseases or conditions, but a method of ensuring that the spine and nervous system is functioning properly by keeping the spine free of spinal subluxations.

Chiropractic has three major components, (1) the science of chiropractic, (2) the art of chiropractic, and (3) the philosophy of chiropractic.

The science of chiropractic is the study and understanding of the human body, but places emphasis on the spine and nervous system.

The art of chiropractic is the knowledge and use of specific spinal adjusting techniques to realign, balance and remove spinal subluxations to keep the spine healthy. There are over 130 different adjusting techniques and some chiropractic techniques are diversified, Gonstead, activator, SOT, and many others. The techniques are delivered by hand to the patient's spine. The style, method, body positions and delivery of a chiropractic adjustment is an art.

The philosophy of chiropractic is based on health and disease which emphasizes two fundamental concepts: (1) the structure and condition of the body influences how the body functions and its ability to heal itself, and (2) the mind-body relationship is instrumental in maintaining health and the healing process.

How does Chiropractic work?

In order to understand how chiropractic works, you first must understand how your body works. Your body is a self-healing and self-regulating organism controlled by your nervous system. Your nervous system begins to form within four hours after conception, and continues to grow and communicate with your body throughout your life. There are over 400 billion bodily instructions transmitted from your brain, into the spinal cord and out to every cell, organ, tissue, and muscle in your body via your nervous system every second of your life. These instructions are then sent back to the brain along the same nervous system pathway to confirm if your body is working properly. Improper motion or position of the spinal bones, called spinal subluxations, can interfere with the nervous system by irritating the nerves, thus causing mis-communication between the brain and body. This can lead to disease, symptoms, pain and even death. It is very similar to talking on your telephone with static on the line. It makes it difficult for the two people to communicate properly. Specific spinal adjustments can remove spinal subluxations, which allow the nervous system to work properly and improve mind and body communications.

How old is the Chiropractic profession?

Early forms of chiropractic treatments have been found dating as far back as 2700 B.C. in China, also in Egypt, India and Greece. The great philosopher Hippocrates (460-370 B.C.), known as the Father of Medicine, talked about spinal misalignments in his books on bones and joints. Hippocrates stated: "Look well to the spine for the cause of disease". Socrates also stated: "If you would seek health, look first to the spine". Findings in early Germany and Scotland suggest they also had a crude type of chiropractor known as a "bone setter". Today's modern form of chiropractic began about 123 years ago in Davenport Iowa.

How was Chiropractic discovered?

Daniel David (D.D.) Palmer (1845-1913) is known as the "discoverer or founder" of chiropractic and was the first to record a chiropractic adjustment on September 18, 1895. He was born in a small town outside of Toronto Canada in 1845. In 1887, he moved to Davenport Iowa and began practicing the art of magnetic healing, a very popular form of healthcare which uses the body's own magnetism to heal. He stumbled upon the theory and discovery of chiropractic after adjusting his buildings janitor, Harvey Lillard, who was deaf at the time and the adjustment restored his hearing. At first, Palmer thought he had discovered a cure for deafness. Shortly after this, he had a patient with heart trouble which was not responding to the magnetic healing. He examined the spine, discovered misaligned vertebrae, gave an adjustment and the patient had immediate relief. He began to reason why two very different diseases came from an impingement of the spinal nerves, were not other diseases due to a similar cause? Thus began the science (knowledge of the human body) and the art (adjusting the spine) of chiropractic.

He opened the Palmer School of Chiropractic in 1897 and by 1902 fifteen people (including five medical doctors and his own 20 year old son, B.J.) had paid the $500 fee and graduated from the 6-month course. In 1906, 24 students had graduated and in 1923, over 3,000 students had graduated. Today, there are more than 10,000 students enrolled in 23 chiropractic colleges in the world.

In 1906, Dr. Palmer and other chiropractors were the first of hundreds of chiropractors to be convicted of practicing medicine without a license. He was jailed, server 23 days, paid a $350 fine and then was released. A year later in Wisconsin, one of his graduates, Dr. Shegataro Morikubo, was arrested for practicing medicine, surgery and osteopathy without a license. However, in a landmark decision, the judge and jury agreed the Morikubo was not practicing medicine, surgery or osteopathy. Rather, he was practicing something different; chiropractic.

From 1906 thru 1913, Dr. Palmer published two books on chiropractic, <u>The Science of Chiropractic</u> and <u>The Chiropractor's Adjuster</u>. Palmer died from a lengthy battle with typhoid fever on October 20, 1913.

What does the word "Chiropractic" mean?

In 1895, after his new health care discovery, Dr. Palmer asked his good friend and patient, Reverend Samuel Weed to help name this new discovery. After careful discussion and research with Dr. Palmer, Reverend Weed came up with the combination of two Greek words; "cheiro" (meaning hand), and "praktikus" (meaning action or to be done by). He put the two words together and interpreted the new word as "to be done by hand" or Chiropractic.

Who was the first Chiropractic patient?

The first chiropractic adjustment was given to an African-American man named Harvey Lillard (1856-1925). As the story is told, Mr. Lillard was the owner of a janitorial service that maintained the building where Dr. Palmer practice his magnetic healing, a hands on therapy which was also practiced by many medical doctors of the 19th century era.

Lillard had told Palmer that he had suffered from both neck and back pain and that he had lost most of his hearing over 17 years before. Lillard added that he could no longer hear sounds like the horses hoofs just out side a window or the ticking of a pocket watch.

Palmer asked Lillard how he had lost his hearing and he replied that while bent over in a stooped position he heard something "pop" in his spine and immediately lost most of his hearing.

Palmer examined Lillard and found a small lump on his back. He recognized this lump as a badly misaligned vertebra and reasoned that since it had occurred when Lillard went deaf; restoring the vertebra to its proper position might also restore his hearing. He presented this theory to Lillard and requested that he be allowed to try and realign the vertebra. Having known Palmer for years, Lillard agreed to let Palmer work on his neck and back.

Palmer felt that Lillard's hearing loss was due to a blockage of the spinal nerves which control the inner ear. This nerve blockage and bone misalignment lessened the body's ability to function properly. When Palmer corrected the misalignment by pushing the vertebra back into place, the nerve pathway was reopened and thus Lillard's hearing was restored.

Who is B.J. Palmer?

Bartlett Joshua (B.J.) Palmer (1881-1961) is the son of Dr. D.D. Palmer and is known as the "developer of chiropractic". B.J. was one of the first to graduate from the Palmer Chiropractic College in 1902 (at age 20), along with 23 other students. In late 1902 while his father was on trial for practicing medicine without a license, B.J. officially took over as President of Palmer College. In 1910, B.J. introduced the world to the use of x-rays as a diagnostic instrument.

B.J. is credited with expanding and researching chiropractic and for making it become mainstream healthcare. He is credited with writing over 40 books, numerous research articles, and teaching at the Palmer College. His last book; Palmer's <u>Law of Life</u> was written in 1958.

In 1924, Palmer had the first radio station west of the Mississippi, WOC (Wonders of Chiropractic). In 1928, he purchased another radio station in Des Moines Iowa, WHO (With Hands Only).

Dr. B.J. Palmer's patients included US Presidents and business leaders from all over the world. Ronald Reagan (one of the first disc jockeys at WOC), magician Harry Houdini, Presidents Herbert Hoover, Harry Truman and Calvin Coolidge, along with boxing great Jack Dempsey and the world famous Barnum and Bailey circus performers were frequent guests in his home.

Who was the first female Chiropractor?

Minora Paxson is credited with being one of the first females to attend and graduate from Palmer College in 1905. After graduation, she was one of the first female faculty members along with Mabel Palmer (B.J.'s Palmers wife). Almeda Haldeman is regarded as the first female chiropractor to practice in Canada, graduating in 1905 and beginning practice in 1906. She also helped her son establish the first Canadian Chiropractic College in Toronto. Another early female graduate, Barbara Brake also graduated in 1905 and returned to Melbourne Australia and opened the first chiropractic college in Australia. Fred Rubel is known as the first African-American chiropractor, graduating from National College of Chiropractic in 1913 and then started his own short lived chiropractic college in 1921.

What is a spinal subluxation?

A spinal subluxation is a condition in which one or more spinal vertebrae (back bones) are out of normal alignment. This places pressure on the spinal nerves and affects the normal transmission of nerve impulses. The function and healing process of vital parts of the body is often affected. Although extreme pain has been observed in some cases, it is more often noticed as a discomfort. If the condition is allowed to go untreated, the body will attempt to help support the subluxated vertebrae but may deform instead. Over a period of time, the area becomes calcified, and the vertebrae will actually begin to change shape. The longer the condition is allowed to go untreated, the less chance there is for a complete recovery. What began as a minor problem or discomfort, may lead to a total destruction of the joint and irreversible damage to the nerves. If detected early, a spinal subluxation may respond well to chiropractic treatments with an excellent chance for a complete and painless recovery.

How do I get spinal subluxations?

There are three basic causes of spinal subluxations; (1) physical trauma, (2) emotional stress, (3) chemical imbalances.

(!) Physical trauma: includes slips and falls, auto accidents, work related injuries, playing sports, moving furniture, carrying a baby and car seat, doing yard work, dancing, falling down the stairs, carrying too many grocery bags, roller skating , wearing the wrong shoes, etc, etc. You get the idea. Trauma does not need to be a dramatic injury for the body to become subluxated. Subluxation due to "activities of daily living" can slowly produce subluxations until it reaches a point where it is irritating the nervous system, thus creating symptoms. These daily micro-traumas take months and even years to produce a subluxation that creates symptoms or pain.

(2) Emotional stress: includes work or home stresses, dealing with the in-laws, divorce, planning a wedding, moving, selling or buying a home, holiday stress, homework, paying the bills or taxes, grief, anger, fear, frustration, depression, etc, etc.

(3) Chemical imbalances: a poor diet, alcohol, soda pop, coffee, over-eating, too much salt or fatty foods, smoking, prescription and non-prescription drug use, illegal drug use, etc.

One, two or even all three may be causing your subluxations, although all three need not be present to create subluxations.

How do I know if I have a spinal subluxation?

It is difficult to tell when you have a subluxation, sometimes you can, but most often you can'. Like the early stages of tooth decay or cancer, spinal subluxations (known as the silent killer) can be present long before pain or other symptoms appear. Our activities of daily living usually bring on subluxations slowly and without any pain or symptoms. Even activities such as sleeping can bring on subluxations. Traumatic injuries, such as car accidents or slip and falls, usually bring them on quickly with symptoms and are very easy to determine.

Can spinal subluxations clear up on their own?

Rarely, but it is not very likely. Today's hectic lifestyles are a constant source of spinal subluxations. Fortunately, our bodies have the ability to self-correct many of these smaller problems as we bend and twist, or stretch. But when our lives become too hectic or we have a serous trauma involved, our bodies begin to shut down and not work properly. Pain is produced and that is when most people present to the chiropractors office, for pain relief. But chiropractic is more than pain relief.

How do I know when I need a Chiropractic adjustment?

If you have never had chiropractic care before, it may be difficult to know when to seek treatment from a chiropractor. A traumatic injury or chronic pain is the usual symptom that prompts a first visit to the chiropractor, but a growing number of people seek chiropractic care to enhance their overall health and well being.

A person's need for chiropractic adjustments varies greatly, depending on their general health, physical condition and age, lifestyle, past health history, injuries, and hereditary factors. But the presence of pain is not necessarily the best indicator that chiropractic adjustments are needed. Once a condition has reached the point of pain, a great deal of damage from the strains and irritation has already occurred.

Some people choose ongoing chiropractic care either to minimize existing conditions or to help prevent future problems from occurring. This may be your best insurance for obtaining and keeping optimum health.

What is an X-ray?

X-rays or radiographs are the use of radiation for different types of imaging of the body, primarily the skeletal system. Radiology is an important part of determining the correct diagnosis and treatment of a patient. Poor imaging of an x-ray or a wrong interpretation can lead to a wrong diagnosis and wrong treatment of a patient's condition. Without x-rays a complete "picture" of the patient is not possible.

Who discovered X-rays?

Wilhelm Roentgen (1845-1923) was a German physicist who discovered x-rays on November 8, 1895. Before his discovery, Dr. Roentgen earned a PhD. Degree in physics from the University of Zurich in 1869. Through his studies and experiment with cathode ray tubes, this led him to the discovery of a new and different kind of ray. Because the nature of these strange rays was then unknown, he gave them the name x-rays (unknown rays). The first x-ray, also called "roentgenogram", ever produced was of his wife's left hand which also shows her wedding ring. In 1901 he won the Novel Prize in Physics for his discovery of the x-ray.

Why do I need X-rays?

Because seeing is knowing and not seeing is guessing. And chiropractors will not guess when it comes to providing the best possible care for their patients. Without actually seeing the positions of the spinal vertebrae, spinal decay and bone spurring, and osteoarthritis, it may cause an inaccurate diagnosis and treatment of your condition. You would not want your auto mechanic to work on your car blindfolded, so why would you allow your chiropractor to not see what is inside of your body?

What is a CAT scan?

Computed Axial Tomography (CAT or CT) scan is the process of using computers to generate a three dimensional image from flat x-ray images, one slice at a time. A large donut shaped x-ray machine takes x-ray images at many different angles around the body. These images are processed by a computer to produce cross sectional pictures of the body. In each of these pictures, the body is seen as an x-ray slice of the body, which is then recorded on film. This recorded image is called a tomogram.

If you were to imagine the body as a loaf of bread and you are looking at one end of the loaf. As you remove each individual slice of bread, you can see the entire surface of that slice from the crust to the center. The body is seen on CT scan slices in a similar way from the skin to the central part of the body. When these levels are further added together, a three dimensional picture of the body can be obtained. This technique is painless and can provide extremely accurate images of the body and the internal organs.

What is an EMG?

An electromyography (EMG) study is usually performed for a chronic pain syndrome, numbness or tingling in the arms or legs. It tests the condition of the nerves from the spine into the arm or leg, and whether those nerves are functioning normal. To test the nerves, mild electrical impulses are sent along the nerve pathway in the arm or leg and measured against a "normal" finding. The intensity of the impulses will be slowly increased until a response occurs. The electrical impulses will make the muscles "jump and twitch", and will feel much like a static electrical shock. This test can be slightly uncomfortable for some people, so it is best to discuss the test and what it entails thoroughly with your neurologist.

What is a Chiropractic adjustment?

The main treatment method used by chiropractors is the "chiropractic manipulative therapy" also known as the chiropractic adjustment. It is a specific procedure using carefully directed and controlled pressure, usually done by hand, to restore spinal bones to a more normal position and have proper motion. In technical terms, it is the act of moving the spinal joints beyond the normal physiological range of motion using a high speed, low amplitude thrust. This generates a release within the joint which may cause a loud popping noise (an audible) as the movement takes place. The adjustment consists of placing the patient on a specially designed adjusting table and applying pressure, using specialized techniques, to the areas of the spine that are subluxated. There are over 125 different adjusting techniques in use by chiropractors today.

How many adjustments do I need?

The specific number of adjustments varies with each individual patient and their individual health care goals (pain relief, corrective care, or preventive care). Many patients notice progress within a week or two with frequent visits. Each adjustment builds on the previous adjustment. Missing appointments makes your adjustments less effective and allows your condition to continue to progress. Visits become less often as your spine begins to stabilize and your health improves. In chronic cases, complete healing and recovery may take several months or even years.

How should I feel after an adjustment?

How you feel depends on you. Some people feel great and have immediate results, while others may be slightly sore. Still others may feel no change at all. The majority of patients do feel some type of soreness in the area they received the adjustment, but the soreness can be relieved with a short treatment of ice or heat therapy, rest or even massage. That is why it is essential to communicate all changes in your symptoms, good or bad, with your chiropractor so he can modify your treatment accordingly. Whenever you begin a new endeavor, whether it is chiropractic, stretching or exercise, the initial shock to your body will always cause some discomfort. Don't stop your treatments prematurely due to the soreness. It will get better with

time and as your body becomes more accustomed to the
adjustments.

How come I have to come back so many times?

Many patients visit the chiropractor due to some
type of chronic pain syndrome, which is a condition
which had progressively worsened over time. The
adjustments build on one another until the patients
condition has stabilized and is pain-free. It is very
similar to dieting or working out at the gym. You don't
diet one day a month and expect to lose weight or
workout once a month and expect to build and tone
your muscles. Each activity builds upon the other. The
more problematic your condition, the longer you have
had your condition, and the current treatment which
you are receiving all play into how often you need to
have adjustments. The longer and more severe your
condition, the longer it may take to correct and stabilize
it. Only your chiropractor can determine your treatment
plan and what necessary steps it will take to correct
your spinal condition.

What happens if the adjustments don't work for me?

If your chiropractor is unable to find and correct the
cause of your particular spinal problem, he will refer
you to other specialists who may be able to help you.
Other specialists may include an orthopedist,

neurologist, nutritionist, massage therapists, physical therapist, etc, etc. Your chiropractor is dedicated to getting you as well as he can and as fast as he can. And if that means referring you to another physician, he will. Your health is his main concern.

How old should I be when I get my first adjustment?

There is no specific age when you should receive your first adjustment or when you should receive your last. Many people begin some type of chiropractic care in their mid-twenties when some type of injury occurs. Others (like myself) began receiving care soon after birth and continue with some type of ongoing treatment throughout their life. I still find it amazing when a new patient begins care well into their fifties with serious trauma throughout their life, and never having been to a chiropractor and expect their spinal conditions to clear up in one or two treatments. Years of neglect, abuse and spinal decay have developed and it will take time to correct those conditions.

Are all patients adjusted the same?

No. Every patient's spinal condition and health history is different and therefore each chiropractic treatment plan is individualized to that specific patient. Chiropractors see a wide variety of spinal subluxations and distortions and to treat every patient the same would be dangerous and foolish. For example, a 25 year old aerobics instructor who wants regular, preventive care and the 35 year old pregnant mom of 3 children and a 60 year old male "retired couch potato" who was involved in a car accident would not have the same treatment plan. Each patient's treatment plan is custom-tailored for their age, health conditions, and injury and health care goals.

Can I adjust myself?

No. Although some people cam make their joints "pop and snap", it may sound like an adjustment but it is not a chiropractic adjustment. Even worse, damage can occur to a joint which results in weakened muscles and ligaments. Adjustments are very specific and take years of training and practice to master. Even your chiropractor can not adjust himself and must visit their own chiropractor to receive adjustments.

Do I have to take my clothes off to get adjusted?

No. Maybe. Yes, but not always. It depends on the type of adjusting technique your particular chiropractor is using to treat your condition. But most chiropractors do require you change into wearing a gown when receiving a spinal examination or x-rays. Your weekly adjustment usually does not require you to wear a gown or disrobe, but you can keep your street clothes when receiving your adjustment.

Can my spine move too much from an adjustment?

It is very unlikely. Besides, only the spinal joints that are subluxated receive adjustments. This allows the weakened muscles and ligaments around the joint to stabilize and heal. A chiropractic adjustment is very specific and deliberant. It has the right amount of energy, delivered to an exact spot, at a precise angle, at just the right time. The intent is to get a "stuck" vertebrae moving again, helping to reduce nerve interference. Years of training, practice and experience make adjustments specific and safe.

How long will it take to get better?

There are many, many factors that determine the amount of time it takes a patient to have relief. Some patients experience almost instant relief. Others discover it may take a few days, and others can take many weeks or months depending on your specific condition. Within a short period of time, most patients can feel a change progressing through their body to fully carry out their chiropractor's treatment plan recommendations.

Are there any famous people that visit the Chiropractor?

Yes! Many, many television and movie stars, all-star athletes, politicians and other celebrities use chiropractic. Some names you may recognize include: Burt Reynolds, Anthony Robbins, Tom Brady, Kareem Abdul-Jabbar, Mel Gibson, Sylvester Stallone, Jerry Seinfeld, Richard Gere, Madonna, Whoopie Goldberg, Arnold Schwarzenegger, Clint Eastwood, Michael Jordan, Tiger Woods and the list goes on and on. Over 55 million Americans visit a chiropractor every year.

Why do newborns and infants need to be adjusted?

Preliminary studies suggest that infantile colic, unusual crying, poor appetite; ear infections or erratic sleeping habits can be signs of spinal subluxations caused by the birthing process or by the position of the fetus in the womb. Pediatric adjustments are very gentle and very safe. Knowing exactly where to adjust, the chiropractor applies no more pressure than you would use to test the ripeness of a tomato to make the adjustment.

How can I prevent getting spinal subluxations?

Due to the various stresses in our daily lives, it is very difficult to prevent getting subluxations. As previously mentioned, daily activities play a major role of stress and strain on our bodies, and sometimes our bodies can handle those stresses, and other times it can't. The best prevention is to watch what you eat, exercise daily, control your weight, and receive regular scheduled adjustments.

Will I ever be normal again?

"Normal" is a relative term and it has different meanings to different people. Chiropractic results vary from patient to patient. Many people report improved spinal curves, spinal motion and the total resumption of their normal lifestyles. Those who neglected or delayed seeking care often see slower progress. After improvement, many patients discover that periodic chiropractic adjustments can help avoid a relapse of their conditions.

Does my health insurance cover Chiropractic services?

Yes! Under the Every Category of Provider law, insurance companies are required by laws to provide chiropractic health benefits. Most insurance covers basic care for chiropractors, but not long term corrective care. Some health insurance limits you to a specific dollar amount or a specific number of office visits per year. Either way, you should not judge your need for treatment on your insurance coverage. Don't depend on your insurance coverage to provide all the needed and necessary treatment needed to correct your condition.

Are Chiropractors "real doctors"?

Absolutely! Following high school graduation, a minimum of a four year college education earning a bachelors degree, and then continuing on to a chiropractic college for an additional four years must be completed to earn the degree of Doctor of Chiropractic (D.C.).

Are Chiropractic adjustments safe?

Chiropractic has an excellent safety record. In the words of the New Zealand governments inquire; chiropractic care is "remarkably safe". By avoiding harmful prescription drugs and over the counter drugs with their long list of side effects, and risky surgery, chiropractic enjoys an excellent track record. Comparing the statistics, adjustments are about 100 times safer than taking an over the counter pain reliever. And if that is not clear enough, you have a better chance of winning the lottery than getting injured by a chiropractic adjustment.

How effective are Chiropractic adjustments?

In recent years, advances in chiropractic techniques and research studies have shown quite dramatically that chiropractic care may be the preferred approach to the management of soft tissue injuries. Pain and decreased joint mobility are among the most commonly seen chronic complaints following an automobile accident.

Clinical studies have repeatedly demonstrated the value of spinal manipulation for the restoration of normal neck functioning.

In 1944, the National Chiropractic Association (NCA) created the Chiropractic Research Foundation (CRF) with the objective of promoting and acquiring funding for the development of research for the chiropractic profession.

A 1986 orthopedic study indicated that early utilization of exercise and spinal mobilization is superior to the traditional treatment of soft tissue injuries for the tested factors of pain reduction and increased mobility.

In 1990, the British Medical Journal reported on the findings of a ten year study comparing chiropractic with out-patient hospital care of patients suffering from acute and chronic low back pain. The researchers found a significant, reliable, and measurable advantage for chiropractic treatment over conventional hospital out-patient management of back pain. The authors of this study concluded that patients treated by chiro-practors fared considerably better in their recovery.

Today, chiropractic research continues to grow and much credit is due to the assistance of a number of other organizations within the chiropractic profession. The scope of chiropractic research parallels that of medical research, with active research in such areas as basic sciences, health services, education and clinical research.

Are there different ways to be adjusted?

Yes. There are over 130 different adjusting techniques to adjust the spine. Each technique has its own specific design and reasoning why that technique should be used on a particular patient. Your chiropractor has been trained in many different techniques, and the one he uses on you depends entirely on your specific needs and conditions.

What is that popping sound I hear when I get adjusted?

It is the sound of nitrogen gas being released from the spinal joint as it returns to the normal position. It is much like opening a bottle of champagne or removing a suction cup. The sound is interesting, but not all adjustments create this sound, so don't rate your adjustment as good or bad depending on the loudness of the pop. Unlike a very common misconception about the popping noise, it is definitely not bones breaking or cracking.

I'm pregnant. Can I still be adjusted or will it harm the baby?

Yes, it is very safe and very sensible for both mother and her baby. What some people don't understand is that today's chiropractic care is beneficial to both the mother and to her baby. Plus, many chiropractors have had special training to use special techniques which help a baby assume the best possible position for a safe delivery. It is generally used when a baby is in a breech position and many women have successfully avoided Caesarean births because of this technique.

Some of the many benefits of chiropractic care during pregnancy include: improved functioning of the nervous system which helps both the mother and the fetus, proper alignment of the pelvis which supports the growing uterus and allows maximum room for the baby to grow, provides proper positioning of the baby for labor and delivery which aids in reducing the amount of pain the mother experiences during labor and allows for an easier birth process, and reduces lower back and pelvic pain due to the added weight of the developing baby.

Why do children go to the Chiropractor?

For the same basic reasons adults do, to get their spines checked for spinal subluxations. By some estimates, more than one in ten adolescent boys an done in five girls suffer from long-term neck and shoulder symptoms. Possible causes range from playing musical instruments to participating in sports to carrying too heavy of a backpack. In one study involving data collected from students in grades 7-9, all of whom were assessed for neck or upper arm pain occurring at least weekly in the preceding six months, upper arm pain appeared almost weekly in nearly one-third of the students.

Interestingly, students were more likely to develop neck and upper arm pain in the period from fall to

spring, as opposed to spring to fall. This aroused
suspicions that carrying heavy backpacks and the
stresses of school were somehow linked to the
symptoms.

How does the education of a Chiropractor and a medical doctor compare?

There are many similarities but also key differences
in both types of education. Both chiropractic and
medical education emphasize knowledge of the basic
sciences such as anatomy, physiology, neurology,
pathology and chemistry. How the human body is
designed and functions is extremely important to both
types of doctors. Chiropractors devote a great deal of
study in the classroom and in practice to the function of
the nervous system and to the structure of the human
body; both of these systems affect the quality of a
person's health and well being. Chiropractic education
also contains increasing study in nutrition as an
important consideration in restoring and maintaining
health of the body. Medical doctors devote more study
to pharmacology and toxicology so that they can
understand how medications and other substances
affect the body relative to conditions that are being
treated.

Both chiropractors and medical doctors must pass
stringent graduation requirements and national and state
board examinations to obtain a license to practice. Even
though traditional chiropractic and medical approaches
for treatment of a patient differ, it is important to note
that there is increasing cooperation among all types of

healthcare providers as they work for the common good of the people seeking care.

Where do you go to college to obtain a Chiropractic degree?

Before you can begin your schooling at a chiropractic college, you must first attain a high school or GED diploma and a bachelor's degree from a four year college. This will then allow you to apply to one of the 33 chiropractic colleges in the world.

There are 18 chiropractic colleges in the United States, with other colleges in Canada, Europe, and Australia. The first chiropractic college was founded in 1897 in Davenport Iowa by Dr. D.D. Palmer. The Palmer Chiropractic College (named after the founder of chiropractic) remains today and is known as the Fountainhead of Chiropractic.

What type of education does a Chiropractor receive?

Since 1974, standards for chiropractic education have been established and monitored by the Council on Chiropractic Education (CCE), a non-profit organization located in Scottsdale Arizona.

Admissions requirements of chiropractic colleges are influenced by the CCE standards and chiropractic licensing board requirements. A minimum of four year bachelors degree is required with successful completion of courses in biology, chemistry, physics, psychology, English and the humanities.

A chiropractic program consists of four academic years of professional education averaging a total of 4,822 hours of course work. Several areas of study are emphasized during the course of chiropractic education: adjustive techniques, spinal analysis, neurology, anatomy and physiology, x-ray technique, microbiology, biochemistry, pathology, orthopedics, diagnosis, bio-mechanics, principles and practice of chiropractic.

The practice of chiropractic is licensed and regulated in all 50 states in the U.S. and in over 30 countries worldwide.

Why should I go to the Chiropractor? I don't have any back pain.

Don't get caught up in the idea that if you have no pain, you must be healthy. Pain is the very last symptom to show up and is the first to go away once treatment has begun. Take for example a person with cancer. When did they become ill with the cancer? When they were diagnosed? Or was it many months or years before while the cancer was growing "under the radar"? Many cancer patients have no pain, but are they healthy? Another example is tooth decay or cavities. When does a person know when a cavity has occurred? When the cavity reaches the nerve and creates pain? Or was it before while it was growing buy was pain free during the process? So why should you go to the Chiropractor? Because an ounce of prevention is worth a pound of cure and having a healthy spinal column and proper working nervous system makes good sense. Regular spinal check ups can help you avoid serious spinal injuries before they occur.

How many licensed Chiropractors are there in the United States?

Currently there are over 100,000 practicing licensed Chiropractors in the world today in over 92 countries.

I was hurt at work. Can I still go to the Chiropractor?

Yes. If you are injured at work and have reported the injury to your supervisor, you may file a claim with Labor and Industries. The department of L&I will cover your expenses associated with the injury.

How come Chiropractors claim to cure everything?

Remember, only the body heals itself. The Chiropractor claims to cure nothing, the patient may be relating other symptoms they suffered from an dare beginning to clear up after receiving adjustments. The Chiropractor only treats the spine and nervous system and when the nervous system is functioning at 100% capacity, without interference, many patients find their chronic symptoms clear up.

How can Chiropractic adjustments help my headaches?

There are many, many different types and causes of headaches. Fortunately, many of these causes can be relieved with chiropractic adjustments. A headache is an alarm signaling a problem in your body. Rather than masking the symptom with over the counter drugs or prescription medication, your chiropractor will treat your headaches by treating its underlying cause.

I've heard that once you start going to the Chiropractor you have to go for the rest of your life. Is that true?

No. Of course not, but many patients choose to continue with some type of periodic, wellness treatment after they get the results they want. Patients receive treatment, get the results they want, and then continue their care in a lesser degree to maintain and control the results they have achieved. It is always your choice on ho long you decide to benefit from chiropractic care.

Do Chiropractors prescribe medications?

No. Chiropractors don't dispense prescription or non-prescription drugs of any kind. Medications only cover up symptoms and do nothing to correct the cause of those symptoms. While chiropractors make no use of drugs or surgery, chiropractors do refer patients for medical care when those who need medicine and surgery are necessary.

Why do medical doctors and Chiropractors not get along?

For many years there was quite a misunderstanding between the medical doctors and chiropractors, but that's changing. Years of prejudice and bias are giving way to research showing the benefits of chiropractic care. Attitudes are slowly changing. More and more medical doctors are accepting what chiropractors can do for their patients, and referrals have become more commonplace now.

I was involved in a motor vehicle accident recently. The doctor at the hospital said I have a whiplash injury and should be fine in a few days and prescribed muscle relaxers for me. But I continue to hurt. Is there anything Chiropractic can do for me?

Yes. Motor vehicle collisions injuries are very serious. Each and every motor vehicle collision have different circumstances because of the collision factors and the different physical characteristics of the people involved. Chiropractic treatments of whiplash injuries provides pain relief, removes pressure on nerves, and prevents the growth of spinal arthritis by normalizing the movement of individual segments of the spine.

What is whiplash?

Whiplash is a powerful force, like the sudden sharp snap of a whip, it hurls your head backwards and forward injuring you neck. A car accident, sports injury, or simply a sudden, unexpected push from behind can create a whiplash. Chiropractors are pine specialists uniquely trained to diagnose and treat whiplash injuries, relieve its symptoms and help prevent more serious injuries from developing.

What is the difference between a sprain and a strain?

A sprain is an injury to the *ligaments* around a joint (think of a sprained ankle), while a strain is an over-stretching or over exertion of the *muscles* of the body.

What is a slipped disc?

A "slipped disc" is a common way, although incorrect way, to refer to a wide variety of spinal disc problems. However, a disc can't slip out of position because of the way it attaches to the spinal bones above and below it. It can tear, bulge, dry out, thin out and it can also become herniated and collapse, but it can not slip out of place.

What is a disc tear?

The most common disc injury is a small crack or micro-tear in the tough, outer cartilage material of the disc called the annular fibers. This small tear allows the soft jelly in the middle of the disc to start leaking out, and the disc begins to wear thin. This is often painless until the soft center of the disc finds its way out along the cracks and tears of the disc and produces pressure on the spinal nerve root.

What is a bulging disc?

The spinal disc is a small cartilage pad that is situated between two spinal bones. The soft jelly-like center is contained by layers of tough fibrous tissues. Each disc serves as connector, space, and shock absorber for the spine. The discs are much thicker in your low back region than in your neck because of the added weight of the body placed upon the spine. When healthy, discs allow normal turning and bending.

The soft jell-like material in the middle of the disc pushes to one side, forward or backward, and swelling occurs. The middle is still contained within the tough outer fibers of the disc, but can still cause pressure and painful symptoms.

What is a herniated disc?

The soft jelly-like material from the center of the spinal disc ruptures through the tough, outer fibers and extends to the outer edge or beyond the normal limits of the disc. A MRI is the diagnostic tool of choice for determining if the patient has a herniated or other treatment. Many times the only treatment option is surgery to correct the herniated disc.

What is spinal stenosis?

Spinal stenosis is a narrowing of spaces in the spine that result in pressure on the spinal cord and the nerve roots. The narrowing may involve a small or large area of the spine. This disorder is very common in men and women over 50 years of age. However, it may occur in younger people who are born with a narrowing of the spinal canal or who suffer an injury to the spine.

What is scoliosis?

The word "scoliosis" comes from the Greek language and translates into "a lateral or abnormal deviation from center." Scoliosis primarily affects children and is difficult to detect because children rarely complain of any pain. But some of the classic signs that a child is developing scoliosis are: one shoulder is higher than the other, one hip is higher than the other, the head is tilted to one side, and one shoulder blade flares out more than the other. Chiropractic offers tremendous potential in the management and ongoing monitoring of scoliosis, particularly in its early stages.

What is sciatica?

Sciatica is defined as a pain along the large sciatic nerve that runs from the lower back down the back of each leg. It is a fairly common form of low back and leg pain. This pain along the sciatic nerve can be caused when a nerve root in the spine is pinched or irritated by subluxated lumbar spinal vertebrae. Sciatica responds very well to chiropractic adjustments, primarily to the lumbar spine and pelvis.

What is referred pain?

Referred pain is a very common condition. It is defined as pain from a malfunctioning or disease area of the body, perceived in another area, often far from the origin. A common example is found in a person having a heart attack. They often complain of pain down the left arm and forearm and up into the face, when the origin of the pain is in the chest. Another example is the gall bladder referring pain into the right shoulder. The important fact is to remember that where there is pain in these and other areas, it may indicate a hidden problem which must be found and corrected.

What is degenerative disc disease?

Degenerative disc disease (DDD) also known as degenerative joint disease (DJD) is one of the most common causes of low back pain and also one of the most misunderstood conditions. Many patients diagnosed with low back pain caused by DDD are confused about this diagnosis and what it exactly means to them. Part of the confusion lies within the fact that DDD is not a disease and is not a life threatening condition. DDD is a degenerative process that at times can cause low back pain from a decaying and damaged spinal disc. Disc degeneration is a natural part of aging and over time all people will have some form of degeneration in their discs, depending on the amount of trauma that particular person has had in their lifetime. However, not all people will develop symptoms associated with DDD. Some common names associated with DDD are osteoarthritis, spinal decay and bone spurs.

I have been diagnosed with arthritis. Can I still be adjusted or will it make my arthritis worse?

There are many different types of arthritis, including rheumatoid arthritis, but the most common form is called degenerative arthritis (osteoarthritis). OA is an abnormal 'wear and tear" form of arthritis. If you've been diagnosed with OA, you can reduce your arthritic symptoms when you make a few dietary and lifestyle changes. Medical treatment of OA is typically restricted to aspirin and other non-steroidal anti-inflammatory drugs, cortisone shots and if necessary, surgery. Chiropractic adjustments will also help you deal with the pain and motion restrictions associated with OA. Light exercise including walking, swimming, yoga, and light impact aerobics are also beneficial. Reducing your intake of "nightshade" vegetables such as potatoes, tomatoes, eggplant and green peppers will also alleviate the pain and swelling associated with OA.

I've been diagnosed with osteoporosis (brittle bone disease). Can I still receive chiropractic adjustments or will it break my bones?

Of course you can go to the chiropractor! When developing a treatment care plan your chiropractor considers the unique circumstances of each individual patient. There are many different techniques to adjust the spine without causing harm or injury to the patient. All chiropractors live by the credence, "first do no harm". The specific adjusting technique used by your chiropractor will be the technique that is best suited to fit your conditions, age, lifestyle and spinal structure.

What is Fibromyalgia?

Fibromyalgia (FM) is a chronic, soft tissue disorder which derives its name from the pain that its sufferers have in their muscles, tendons and ligaments (fibrous tissues). While this grouping of symptoms has been documented for over 100 years, it was not until 1990 that specific diagnostic criteria for this little-understood disorder were developed.

People considered to have FM have widespread pain in combination with tenderness in at least 11 of 18 specific tender point sites on the body. The tender points associated with FM occur in localized areas, particularly the neck, along the spine, shoulders and hips. The disorder's cause remains unknown, and although some believe that trauma or injury that adversely affects the central nervous system may be a factor, as well as changes in muscle metabolism.

Most people find chiropractic adjustments, massage, heat and rest to relieve the symptoms. Chiropractic care is an effective way to provide relief from the pain associated with such conditions.

How do I know when to use heat or ice for an injury?

The application of heat increases the circulation of blood and decrease tension in the muscles. Heat application is advantageous for the relief of chronic muscle tension. It is generally best to apply heat to areas of chronic tension in the absence of recent swelling.

Ice packs applied to the body decreases blood flow, decreases swelling from acute or recent injuries, decreases pain, and increases muscle tension. Application of ice is desirable during periods of acute injury in which strains and sprains have occurred.

It becomes confusing when muscle and ligament tension occurs in the same area as joint swelling. In these instances, it is best to apply heat to the area of muscle tension and ice to the area of swelling. Heat is generally more beneficial for muscle spasms than ice. When unusual or strenuous physical activity is followed by back, neck, shoulder or other joint pain, ice is preferred.

What type of exercise and stretching routine is best for me?

If you have ever watched an infant wake up, you have seen the instinctive movements of twisting, turning, arching of the back, and arm and leg extensions. We all have the inborn urge to stretch our spines and put them in motion as a means of promoting the health of our spine and nervous system. In fact, our spines are built for movement.

There are many, many benefits to exercise including; elevation of your metabolism, reduces muscle tension, decreases your blood pressure, improves your sleep, helps to control or blood sugar levels, increases the good cholesterol (HDL), decreases the triglycerides (fat) in your blood, increases the strength of your bones, makes your heart a more efficient pump, promotes circulation, increases your digestion, helps prevent injuries and strains, and makes you feel healthier and look great.

But in spite of such known benefits, stretching can easily be performed in the wrong way. Many people begin new stretching routines and run into serious problems before too long because they try to accomplish too much too soon. It is essential to work with your chiropractor to develop an exercise routine to improve joint mobility and increase flexibility. Proper exercise and stretching provides too many benefits to not be used daily.

I've heard Chiropractors only treat back pain. Is that true?

No. Many people begin care with a chiropractor because of neck or back pain, but chiropractors treat the spine and nervous system only. Chiropractors do not treat headaches, neck pain, low back pain, etc. although those symptoms are usually why a person seeks out chiropractic care. Chiropractic treatments of spinal subluxations that have been detected in your spine are your chiropractor's area of expertise. Chiropractors are known as "bad back doctors", but that is due to the fact that chiropractic patients usually present with some type of "back ache" that is not responding to traditional medicine. Chiropractors are spine and nervous system specialists.

I'm under a medical doctor's care. Can I still go to the Chiropractor?

Yes! Having your spinal column checked is important no matter what other care you are receiving. Your chiropractor will work with your medical doctor in the treatment of your condition. Communication with both doctors will allow each doctor to perform at their best to deliver the most beneficial treatment for you.

I had neck and back surgery a few years ago and my back still hurts. What can a Chiropractor do for me now?

A chiropractor can not undo what the surgery has done, but it can often help relieve your pain and may help prevent the need for future surgeries. You can be sure that your chiropractor will avoid the surgical area of your spine. Surgery often causes instability above and below the surgical site and this will be the focus of your chiropractic care.

Are there different types of Chiropractic care?

Yes. In fact, there are three very different types of chiropractic care.

(1) Acute care, also known as pain relief care. This type of treatment focuses on the patient's pain symptoms only, such as headaches, neck pain, back pain, etc. This type of care is for the temporary relief of pain and discomfort secondary to spinal subluxations. Acute care would be similar to taking an aspirin which may temporary alleviate your headaches, but it does nothing to correct the cause of your headaches. Putting it another way, it is the same as drying a floor that was getting wet from a leaky roof, but not fixing the leak in the roof. Many times a patient chooses relief care only due to failure to completely understand the benefits of corrective care. Relief care provides temporary relief from your pain and symptoms, but does not correct the problems.

(2) Corrective or reconstructive care. This is the removal or deduction of the cause of your

problems (spinal subluxations), allowing the relief or removal of the symptoms. The other purpose is to slow, stop and reverse the spinal subluxations and the associated spinal decay. Symptoms, although are the first to disappear, are the last stage of a problem. It takes time to eliminate the cause of a problem, but the results are more permanent. Corrective care is necessary not only to relieve or reduce a person's pain or symptoms, but also to remove the actual cause of the problem. Corrective care focuses on making certain the spinal subluxations are gone. Corrective care normally takes anywhere from 6-8 months of treatment. Correcting a patient's spinal structure is similar to pouring liquid Jell-O into a mold. If you remove the mold before the Jell-O hardens, you lose the object you wanted to create. As Jell-O requires time to stabilize, so does your spine.

(3) Wellness or maintenance care. This type of care keeps the body moving forward and helps prevent problems from re-occurring. It is to maintain optimal spinal function which allows the spinal subluxation process and spinal decay to heal rather than worsen under the constant erosion of accumulated uncorrected spinal stress. The treatment plan for this type of care is designed on an individual basis. The end product is ideal health, great energy and life-time health care.

Why do so many people have back problems?

The standard statistic for many years has been that over 80% of all Americans will suffer from back problems at some point in their lifetime. It seems like such an alarming number, but strike up a conversation with several people about back pain and it is easy to understand the magnitude of this situation. Many back problems originate from acute trauma, such as sports injuries, slip and falls, motor vehicle accidents and work place injuries. However, most occur and are caused by poor postural and body movement habits day after day. Look at the children going to school today. With not enough lockers in the schools for book storage, the children must carry heavy backpacks throughout the day. These backpacks can weigh up to as much as 30 pounds! That creates quite an abnormal load on a developing young spine.

Why is my posture so important?

Poor posture can produce some very pronounced effects on your body. As a natural response to postural abnormalities, the body lays down more bone along lines of stress, which can lead to early osteoarthritis, bone spurs, and spinal decay. Slumping can also impact major bodily functions.

Keeping your body balanced and straight, maintaining your neck and back's natural curves and using your back smartly, is a major factor in helping you avoid back injuries and pain. That is why chiropractic puts so much emphasis on proper body mechanics and posture.

How does maintaining a healthy back affect my lifestyle?

It is difficult to determine if maintaining a healthy back adds years to your life, but it can certainly add life to your years. Most chiropractors have personal experience with elderly patients who are able to remain active because they sustain good mobility in their spine and other areas of their bodies, and they make back care a regular part of their entire health program. Achieving and maintaining structural balance, proper spinal alignment, and flexibility are strong deterrents to the accumulation of muscle strains and sprains, that, when left uncared for may eventually wear your body down.

How can Chiropractic help me obtain optimal health and well being?

Optimal health is a state of well being in three distinct areas; physical, mental and social. One of my major goals for maximized living is peace management. A negatively stressful life will not give you a healthy body. A struggling, desperate person will likely experience sickness and disease despite following most of the other important rules of health and wellness. Even if you could be healthy while experiencing stress, you'd just be a healthy miserable person. And who wants that?

On the other hand, someone who has peace of mind, knows who he is, works hard to overcome struggles and experiences loving relationships will very likely enjoy ongoing good health for their entire life. If you are not having a good time living in your body, it is hard for that body to be well or for you to call it healthy. Every felling you have affects some part of your body.

Stress has become a serious health hazard. Celebrations and tragedies alike cause a stress response in the body. Some stress is unavoidable. The only stress-free people on the planet can be visited at any local cemetery. It you don't get a handle on it quick, stress can take a huge toll on your physical, mental and social well-being. Let me share with you the simplest way to turn stress into your ally and not your enemy.

Regular chiropractic adjustments are the quickest and most effective way to reduce stress to your nervous system. Spinal nerve stress, also known as spinal subluxations, is a dangerous mechanism that damages nerves, weakens health and depletes you energy. Many people may walk around with a painless subluxation for years without knowing it. (Review The Big Idea). Chiropractors are the only professionals who specialize in diagnosing and correcting spinal subluxations, the cause of spinal stress, which lead to increased energy, improved health and a rejuvenated body. A subluxated free body will be able to adapt and handle stress, good or bad, on a much better basis than a body full of subluxations.

So, the key to having optimal health and well being is; get regular chiropractic adjustments, eat a good, balanced diet, get plenty of rest and exercise, meditate daily, read positively enforced books, and surround yourself with positive people.

Chapter 5

Did you know…?

…there are 33 chiropractic colleges throughout the world, including the United States (16), Canada, Australia and Europe.

…your foot has 26 bones that are linked together with 33 joints.

…about every 7 years the bones in your skeletal system have been replaced and you have a "new" skeleton.

…a recent health survey found that 39% of adults are at least 10% overweight, 37% exercise regularly, 30% average only 6 hours of sleep at night, 60% drink alcoholic beverages and 31% use tobacco products.

…there are over 30 million Fibromyalgia sufferers in the United States.

…that 20% of the population have a bulging disc without experiencing any symptoms.

…the National Health Interview Survey indicates over 4.4 million Americans were injured in car accidents in 2015 with 38,300 deaths.

…a mouse, a human and a giraffe have the same number of neck (cervical) bones. All mammals have 7 cervical vertebrae!

…blood travels more than 60,000 miles each day through your body.

…the average man has 66 pounds of muscle and 3 pounds of brains.

…graphospasm is the medical term for writer's cramp.

…every organ in your body is connected to the one under you hat.

…your nervous system begins to form 4 hours after conception.

…second hand smoke is the third leading cause of preventable death in the U.S.

…the average adult has 10-12 pints of blood in their body.

…the human body contains 206 bones and over 600 muscles.

…for work-related back injuries, workers are able to get back to work quicker and less expensively when given chiropractic care over traditional medical care.

…a recent Gallop poll of American adults found that 89% experience back pain at least once per month.

…the average brain weighs about 3 pounds, but more than 2 pounds of that is water.

…regular users of aspirin and ibuprofen are twice as likely as non-users to develop chronic acid reflux.
…former Governor Arnold Schwarzenegger praised the chiropractic profession by saying: "Chiropractic is about health and fitness. Chiropractic is about natural, preventive health care. I have experienced this for the last 30 years myself on my own body."

…your heart pumps about 2.5 gallons of blood per minute.

…up to 60% of children will experience back or neck pain by the time they reach age 18.

…in an average 24 hour period, your lungs will use about 3,000 gallons of air.

…garlic is a natural anti-biotic. In fact, garlic oil drops placed directly in the ears helps fight off childhood ear infections.

…there are over 3 trillion (3,000,000,000,000), that's 3 million, million, channels of communication that run to and from the brain through the spinal cord in your neck.

…daily cigarette smokers experience back pain twice as often as non-smokers.

…your heart is about the same size as you clenched fist, weighs approximately 10 ounces and beats about 75 times per minute.

…when you blink an eye, you move over 200 muscles.

…your entire spinal cord weighs less than 4 ounces.

…borborygmus is the medical term for hunger pains.

…you breathe in about 7 quarts of air every minute.

…your fingernails grow four times as fast as your toenails.

…on the average, a smoker loses 11 minutes of their total lifespan for every cigarette smoked.

…your sciatic nerve is approximately the same size as your thumb.

…the bird flu vaccine killed 12 times as many people as the bird flu did!

…it takes 65 muscle to frown and only 13 to smile.

…the first state to license chiropractors was Arkansas in 1915, and the last state was Louisiana in 1974.

…there are over 65,000 licensed, practicing chiropractors in the United States.

…66% of your body is water. Bones are 25% water and human blood is 83% water.

…your nerve impulses travel at over 390 feet per second (that's equivalent to over one entire football field).

…a sneeze can travel at a speed in excess of 100 miles per hour.

…the human body has nine layers of muscle in the back.

…right now, there are about 500 different species of bacteria living in your mouth.

…if you stretched all your veins and arteries in your body end to end, they would stretch out to over 12,000 miles.

…there are 31 pairs of spinal nerve roots extending from the spinal column.

…Hippocrates (460-377 BC), the father of medicine, once said, "Get knowledge of the spine, for this is the requisite for many diseases."

…medical doctors in the United States write over six billion drug prescriptions per year, which equals out to be about 3 prescriptions for every man, woman, and child in the country.

…one drop of blood contains over 5 million red blood cells and over 7,000 white blood cells.

…more than 6,000 children are treated in hospital emergency rooms each year due to school back packs that are too heavy for the child.

…arthritis is not a normal ageing condition, but rather a slow, abnormal decaying process of the bones and joints.

…your hand contains 27 individual bones.

…your body is about 66% water, whereas a jellyfish is about 95% water.

…over 25 million people in the U.S. have osteoporosis (brittle bone disease).

…the largest bone in the human body is the femur (thigh bone).

…the largest organ in your body is your skin, and weighs on the average about 6 pounds.

…80% of your entire nervous system is located in your head (it's your brain).

…alcoholic beverages do not calm your nerves, but over excites them.

…exercise sends natural pain killers flowing through your body.

…an estimated 15-20% of the male population and 25-20% of the female population suffer from migraine headaches.

…your body produces over 10,000 cancer cells per month. But your immune system destroys them.

…the mornings are the toughest part of the day for those with osteoarthritis, as they are forced to move in slow motion until they limber up.

…pain has a purpose. It is a protective mechanism that lets your body know that something is wrong.
(Pain = Pay Attention Inside Now).

…your intestinal tract contains over 400 types of good bacteria.

…on average, you must walk 10 miles to burn off the calories from one Big Mac hamburger (approximately 860 calories).

…men who eat more than four servings of cruciferous vegetables (cauliflower, broccoli, etc.) per week, had a 41% decreased risk of prostate cancer over those men who ate less than four servings per week.

…the thinnest skin in your body is on your eyelids.

…without your fingerprints, it would be very hard to hold onto anything.

…humans have about 80,000 genes in their DNA.

…your heart will beat more than 2.5 billion times in your lifetime.

…red food is good for your heart and blood.

…green foods are natural cancer cell killers.

…the risk of being injured by a chiropractic adjustment is 6 million to 1. Which means you would have to visit the chiropractor once per week for 1,430 years before you were injured!

…780,000 people die from hospital, medical and medication errors every year.

…regular chiropractic patients have a 200% stronger immune system than those who don't receive chiropractic care.

…blondes have more hair than dark-haired people (really, this is not a blonde joke).

Chapter 6

The Pain Questionnaire

The Pain Questionnaire is a simple tool to help you objectively measure the severity of your pain. By taking this questionnaire on a monthly or bi-monthly basis, it can provide an objective measure of your progress.

To take this questionnaire, simply choose which statement is most true for you in each section. Choosing between statements can sometimes be difficult, especially if you suffer from intermittent pain. If this is the case with you, select the question that most accurately describes the general level of discomfort you have experienced over the previous two weeks.

Once you have finished answering all the questions, you can score your questionnaire by adding up the numbers for each of the statements you chose and plotting them on the chart at the end of the chapter.

General Disability from Pain

Sleeping

0   I have no pain when I sleep and am able to sleep well.
1   I have no pain when I sleep, but have disrupted sleep.
2   I have pain, but it does not interfere with my sleep.
3   I am frequently awakened by pain, but am able to sleep for at least six hours.
4   I lose more than three hours of sleep per night due to pain.
5   I am completely unable to sleep due to pain.

Housework Activities

0   I am able to perform any housework without pain.
1   I am able to perform any housework, but it causes a mild increase in pain.
2   I am able to perform any housework, but it causes a moderate increase in pain.
3   I am able to do most light and medium housework due to pain.
4   I am only able to do some light housework due to pain.
5   I am unable to perform any housework due to pain.

Pain Intensity

0   The pain comes and goes and is very mild.
1   The pain is constant and is mild in intensity.
2   The pain comes and goes and is moderate in intensity.
3   The pain is constant and is moderate in intensity.
4   The pain comes and goes and is severe.
5   The pain is constant and is severe.

Changing Degree of Pain

0   The pain is rapidly getting better, or I have no pain.
1   The pain fluctuates, but is definitely getting better.
2   The pain is getting better, but very slowly.
3   The pain is neither improving nor worsening.
4   The pain is gradually worsening.
5   The pain is rapidly worsening.

Medication Use

0   I never use any medications for my pain.
1   I use over the counter medications less than once a month for pain.
2   I use over the counter medications regularly for pain.
3   I use prescription medications less than once per month for pain.
4   I use prescription medications regularly for pain.

5   I use prescription medications daily for pain.

Scoring Your Pain Questionnaire

Add up your total points and mark them on the graph below.

Mild Pain: 0 - 9

Moderate Pain: 10 - 19

Severe Pain: 20 - 25

Chapter 7

The Healthy Lifestyle Questionnaire

The Healthy Lifestyle Questionnaire is a quick and easy way to gauge the overall healthiness of your current lifestyle habits. Next to each statement or question, simply mark the box which most accurately describes you. Once you have finished answering all the questions, you can score your questionnaire by adding up the numbers for each of the statements you chose and plotting them on the chart at the end of this chapter. You can then use this information to look at ways to change some of your unhealthy habits to healthier ones.

How do you rate your own health?
1 Above average.
2 About average.
3 Below average.

How often do you visit a chiropractor?
1 Once every month
2 Only when I need it
3 Rarely or never

How stressful is your day-to-day life?
1 Very low stress.
2 Occasionally stressful.
3 Very stressful.

Are you overweight or underweight?
    1   No.
    2   Yes, by less than 20 pounds.
    3   Yes, by more than 20 pounds.

How often do you take a multi-vitamin?
    1   Every day.
    2   Occasionally.
    3   Rarely or never.

How often do you eat fast food?
    1   Less than once a week.
    2   About once or twice a week.
    3   More than twice a week.

How much pure water do you drink each day?
    1   More than 64 oz.
    2   Between 32 and 64 oz.
    3   Less than 32 oz.

How physically active are you?
    1   Very athletic.
    2   Moderately physically active.
    3   Mildly physically active.

How many miles per week do you run, jog, or walk?
    1   More than five miles.
    2   One to five miles.
    3   Less than one mile.

How often do you stretch your muscles?
    1   Daily
    2   Occasionally
    3   Rarely or never

How often do you participate in recreational sports, such as golf, swimming, tennis, etc?
    1   At least once per week.
    2   About once per month.
    3   Less than once per month.

How often do you use tobacco products?
    1   Rarely or never.
    2   Less than once per week.
    3   At least once per week.

How much alcohol do you consume?
    1   None or very little.
    2   Less than one drink per day.
    3   More than one drink per day.

How many hours of restful sleep do you get each night?
    1   Six to eight hours.
    2   More than nine hours.
    3   Five hours or fewer.

How is your relationship with the person closest to you?
    1   Very satisfied.
    2   Somewhat satisfied.
    3   Unsatisfied.

How satisfied are you with your life right now?
    1   Satisfied.
    2   Somewhat satisfied.
    3   Unsatisfied.

Scoring Your Questionnaire

There is a number next to each answer you checked. Add up these numbers to get your total score.

16 – 24: Excellent Lifestyle Habits. You have a very low risk of developing preventable health conditions.

24 – 32: Good Lifestyle Habits. You have a moderately low risk for developing preventable health conditions.

32 – 40: Borderline Lifestyle Habits. You have a moderately high risk for developing preventable health conditions.

40 – 48: Poor Lifestyle Habits. You are at a high risk for developing preventable health conditions.

Chapter 8

The Thrill of Pills

A row of bottles lined up on my shelf,
It caused me to stop and analyze myself;

One yellow pill in the morning I have to pop,
It goes to my heart so it won't stop.

A little white pill at noon I take,
It goes to my hands so they won't shake.

The pretty blue pills that I use a lot,
They tell me I'm happy when I'm not.

The long purple pill goes to my brain,
Tells me that I'm having a day without pain.

The green round pill tells me not to wheeze,
Or cough or choke or even sneeze.

The tiny red ones, smallest of them all,
They go to my blood so I won't fall.

There is such a colorful array of brilliant pills,
Constantly helping to cure me of all kind of ills.

But what I'd really like to know,
Is what tells each pill where to go!

Chapter 9

Two Chances

You have two chances;
one of getting the germ, and one of not.

And if you get the germ, you have two chances,
one of getting the disease and one of not.

And if you get the disease, you have two chances,
one of dying, and one of not.

And if you die,
you will still have two chances.

Chapter 10

Our Patients Speak

Mary - I was very impressed with Dr. Door and how kind he was. I felt very comfortable.

Beau - Dr. Door is simply the best. The staff is warm and friendly at all times and he is a very caring individual.

Kathy - Dr. Door is an outstanding chiropractor. Not only did he save me from foot surgery for plantar fasciitis, he has also relieved major back issues so I could walk, sit and sleep without pain. He has relieved my shoulder and neck pain as well as relieved my headaches that just would not go away. He does all this with a sense of humor. I always feel better mentally and physically after seeing him.

Jennifer – I came in with my hip in pain. After one adjustment the next day was like a miracle. I could walk with no pain. Dr. Door is the best!

Deborah – If you have not seen Dr. Door you are missing out on the best!

Lily – Dr. Door's adjustments make me feel amazing!

Steven – Great service and a great chiropractor!

Lisa – Our entire family loves going to see Dr. Door and visiting while getting the chiropractic care that we need to live a healthy life. It really makes a difference in our every day life to be aligned properly. Thank you!

Toni - Awesome service!

Amy - Dr. Door is hands down the best chiropractor! I trust him completely and would recommend him highly!

John – I am always treated like family and Dr. Door does amazing work.

Kathleen – Great caring doctor and staff.

Chris – Most excellent care is what I receive from Dr. Door.

Sharon – Dr. Door is very competent and makes me feel great!

Marion - Thanks to Dr. Frank Door and his excellent care I am pain free and no longer needing surgery on my back.

Monica – Great first visit! Friendly staff! Explained things to me very well and took the time to listen to what is going on with my health. Took a genuine interest in what is going on.

Lee - Willows Chiropractic Clinic took my appointment the same day. They were able to help relieve the strain on my back that I have been dealing with for a while. I will be back for sure.

Doreen – Always friendly and they make you feel welcome from the time you walk in the door.

Jeff - Friendly staff, easy to get an appointment especially later in the day. I wouldn't go anywhere else.

David - Dr. Door and his staff made me feel like a million bucks!

Stephanie – I will never be able to thank Dr. Door for everything he has done for me!

Nancy – I had immediate improvement with my headaches with painless treatment.

Ashley - Thanks for keeping me straight!

Joyce – Dr. Door has the 'human touch" and really cares about people.

Patricia – Dr. Door is friendly and very gentle.

Shirley – I would highly recommend Dr. Door to anyone!

Maxine – Dr. Door is number one in my book!

Darrell – The service and people are excellent. They make the patient feel very comfortable and at ease.

Donna – Dr. Door is always upbeat and lively and a lot of fun to visit. Plus he helps ease my back pain.

Lana – Dr. Door has made be feel better than ever!

Jon - Thanks for getting me back on my feet again.

Don – I see Dr. Door for preventative care and I feel great!

Terry – Thanks for giving me back a life free of pain.

Sydney – Dr. Door always hears me; he always has time to listen to my concerns.

Betty – Friendly service, great concern for the patient's health and he has a great staff.

Jim – I almost never have neck pain or headaches thanks to the help from Dr. Door.

Julie – I have been a much healthier person all around since receiving chiropractic care from Dr. Door.

Chapter 11

Chiropractic Colleges

Cleveland Chiropractic College – Kansas City
6401 Rockhill Road
Kansas City, MO 64131
Ph: 800-467-CCKC
www.cleveland.edu

Cleveland Chiropractic College – Los Angeles
590 North Vermont Ave.
Los Angeles, CA 90004
Ph: 800-466-CCLA
www.cleveland.edu

Life Chiropractic College
1269 Barclay Circle
Marietta, GA 30060
Ph: 800-543-3202
www.life.edu

Life-West Chiropractic College
25001 Industrial Blvd.
Hayward, CA 95-4545
Ph: 800-788-4476
www.lifewest.edu

Logan College of Chiropractic
1851 Schoettler Road
Chesterfield, MO 63017
Ph: 800-782-3344
www.logan.edu

National University of Health Sciences
200 East Roosevelt Road
Lombard, IL 60148
Ph: 800-826-6285
www.nuhs.edu

New York Chiropractic College
2360 State Route 89
Seneca Falls, NY 13148
www.nycc.edu

Northwestern College of Chiropractic
2501 West 84th
Bloomington, MN 55431
Ph: 952-888-4777
www.nwhealth.edu

Palmer College of Chiropractic
1000 Brady St.
Davenport, IA 52803
Ph: 563-884-5000
www.palmer.edu

Palmer College of Chiropractic - Florida
4777 City Center Parkway
Port Orange, FL 32129
Ph: 866-585-9677
www.palmer.edu/pccf

Palmer College of Chiropractic – West
90 East Tasman Drive
San Jose, CA 95134
Ph: 800-442-2276
www.palmer.edu/pccw

Parker Chiropractic College
2500 Walnut Hill Lane
Dallas, TX 75229
Ph: 800-438-6932
www.parkercc.edu

Sherman College of Straight Chiropractic
PO Box 1452
Spartanburg, SC 29304
Ph: 800-849-8771
www.sherman.edu

Texas Chiropractic College
5912 Spencer Highway
Pasadena, TX 77505
Ph: 800-468-6830
www.txchiro.edu

Western States Chiropractic College
2900 NE 132nd Ave.
Portland, OR 97230
Ph: 800-641-5641
www.wschiro.edu

About the Author

Dr. Frank J. Door is a second generation chiropractor and was born in Davenport Iowa while his father was preparing to graduate from Palmer Chiropractic College. He received his first chiropractic adjustment at the tender age of 3 days old from Dr. B.J. Palmer and has been under chiropractic care ever since.

His family soon moved back to Puyallup where he was raised on Puyallup's South Hill and graduated from Gov. John R. Rogers High School. In March 1988, he began his chiropractic education at the prestigious Palmer College of Chiropractic-West in Sunnyvale California. He graduated in the spring of 1991, returned home to Puyallup and began private practice and in 1993 he opened Willows Chiropractic Clinic. In 1994, Dr. Door received his post-graduate certification in the diagnosis and treatment of whiplash injuries from the Spine Research Institute of San Diego. In 1996, he received another post-graduate certification as a chiropractic sports physician. He continues to be active in his profession as an upstanding member of the Washington State Chiropractic Association (WSCA).

Dr. Door is very active in his community with local sponsorships of the Puyallup Daffodil parade float, Salvation Army winter coats for kids' drives, Puyallup Food Bank, Emergency Food Network, St. Francis House and many other charitable groups.

Dr. Door and his wife, Julie, and their two children, Brianna and T.J. live on Puyallup's South Hill. His interests include family time, Seahawk and Husky football, Mariner baseball, classic cars and traveling. He also writes children's books in his spare time.

Dr. Door is available to speak to your health fair, civic group, high school career day, science fairs and elementary classrooms at no cost.

Please contact Dr. Door at:

Willows Chiropractic Clinic
PO Box 731268
Puyallup, WA. 98373
Ph: 253-841-6482
Fax: 253-864-0148

E-mail: drdoor@comcast.net

Website: www.drdoor.com